The Reset Way

The 5-Stage Reset for Holistic Wellness

The HealthSpan Institute

The Reset Way:
The 5-Stage Reset for Holistic Wellness

ISBN: 9798323930593

Printed in the United States of America

Contents

Chapter 4:
Stage 1–Leg Compression

Chapter 5:
Stage 2–Whole Body Red Light Therapy

Chapter 6:
Stage 3–Sauna

Chapter 7:
Stage 4–Cold Plunge

Chapter 8:
Stage 5–Jacuzzi

Chapter 9:
Creating Your Personal Reset Routine

Chapter 10:
Complementary Practices for Optimal Results

Chapter 11:
Transforming Your Life with the Reset Way

Conclusion

Appendices

Foreword

In today's fast-paced world, we often find ourselves caught up in the relentless demands of daily life. Stress, anxiety, and neglect of our physical and mental well-being have become all too common. As a result, many of us feel overwhelmed, disconnected, and yearning for a way to restore balance and vitality to our lives.

This is where "The Reset Way" comes in. Based on the groundbreaking approach developed by Reset: Mind and Body, this book offers a powerful and transformative solution to the challenges of modern living. By harnessing the science-backed benefits of the 5-stage reset – leg compression, whole body red light therapy, sauna, cold plunge, and jacuzzi – you can unlock your body's innate potential for healing, rejuvenation, and resilience.

As someone who has personally experienced the profound benefits of the Reset Way, I can attest to its ability to transform lives. Through this book, you'll gain a deep understanding of the science behind each stage of the reset, as well as practical guidance on how to integrate these practices into your own life. Whether you're seeking relief from chronic stress, improved physical performance, or simply a greater sense of overall well-being, the Reset Way offers a clear and compelling path forward.

But this book is more than just a guide to the 5-stage reset. It's a call to action – an invitation to prioritize your own self-care and embrace a new way of living. By committing to the Reset Way, you'll not only experience immediate benefits, but also lay the foundation for a lifetime of optimal health and vitality.

So, if you're ready to take control of your well-being and unlock your full potential, I invite you to dive into the pages of this book with an open mind and a willingness to transform. The Reset Way is more than just a wellness practice – it's a journey of self-discovery and empowerment that can change your life in ways you never thought possible.

Let this book be your guide, your companion, and your source of inspiration as you embark on this remarkable journey. Welcome to the Reset Way.

Kurt A. Richardson, PhD

Introduction

The Importance of Self-Care and Wellness

In today's fast-paced and increasingly demanding world, self-care and wellness have become more crucial than ever before. The constant pressure to succeed, coupled with the endless distractions and stressors of modern life, can take a heavy toll on our physical and mental well-being. When we neglect our own needs and prioritize external demands over our personal health, we risk burnout, chronic stress, and a host of other negative consequences.

However, by making self-care a non-negotiable part of our daily routine, we can build a strong foundation for overall wellness and resilience. Self-care encompasses a wide range of practices, from exercise and healthy eating to stress management and mindfulness. By taking intentional steps to nurture our bodies and minds, we can improve our energy levels, boost our immune function, enhance our cognitive performance, and cultivate a greater sense of overall well-being.

The importance of self-care extends beyond just the individual level. When we prioritize our own wellness, we are better equipped to show up fully in our personal and professional lives. We have more energy and focus to devote to our relationships, our work, and our passions. By modeling the importance of self-care, we can also inspire others to prioritize their own well-being, creating a ripple effect of positive change in our communities and beyond.

Overview of Reset: Mind and Body's Approach

Reset: Mind and Body is a company that has pioneered a unique and holistic approach to wellness. Founded on the belief that optimal health requires a comprehensive and integrated approach, Reset has developed a groundbreaking system that combines cutting-edge therapies and ancient wisdom to help individuals achieve their full potential.

At the core of Reset's approach is the recognition that true wellness involves a balance of physical, mental, and emotional factors. Rather than focusing on just one aspect of health, Reset takes a whole-person approach that addresses the interconnectedness of the body and mind. By combining a range of therapeutic modalities, including compression therapy, light therapy, thermal therapy, and more, Reset aims to promote healing, recovery, and overall vitality.

One of the key principles of Reset's approach is the importance of consistency and commitment. While the 5-stage reset can provide immediate benefits, the true power of the Reset Way lies in making these practices a regular part of one's lifestyle. By committing to a consistent self-care routine, individuals can experience profound and lasting improvements in their health and well-being.

Brief Description of the 5-Stage Reset

The Reset Way is anchored by a powerful 5-stage reset that combines the most effective and scientifically-validated therapies for promoting healing, recovery, and overall wellness. The five stages are as follows:

1. Leg Compression: Using specialized compression garments or devices, this stage helps to improve circulation, reduce swelling, and promote lymphatic drainage in the lower body.

2. Whole Body Red Light Therapy: This stage involves exposure to red and near-infrared light, which has been shown to stimulate cellular energy production, reduce inflammation, and promote tissue repair.

3. Sauna: The use of heat therapy through sauna sessions has been shown to improve cardiovascular function, boost immune response, and promote detoxification.

4. Cold Plunge: Exposure to cold temperatures, such as through a cold plunge pool, can help to reduce inflammation, improve

mental clarity, and boost the body's natural healing processes.

5. Jacuzzi: The final stage of the reset involves immersion in a
warm water jacuzzi, which can help to relax muscles, reduce
stress, and promote a sense of overall well-being.

By combining these five stages into a comprehensive reset, the
Reset Way provides a powerful tool for optimizing physical and
mental health. Whether used as a standalone practice or integrated into a larger self-care routine, the 5-stage reset offers a simple
and effective way to promote healing, recovery, and overall wellness.

References

1. Kiecolt-Glaser, J. K., & Wilson, S. J. (2017). Lovesick: How couples' relationships influence
health. Annual Review of Clinical Psychology, 13, 421-443.
2. Laukkanen, J. A., Laukkanen, T., & Kunutsor, S. K. (2018). Cardiovascular and other health
benefits of sauna bathing: a review of the evidence. Mayo Clinic Proceedings, 93(8),
1111-1121.
3. Shui, S., Wang, X., Chiang, J. Y., & Zheng, L. (2015). Far-infrared therapy for cardiovascular,
autoimmune, and other chronic health problems: A systematic review. Experimental
Biology and Medicine, 240(10), 1257-1265.

Part I: The Science Behind the Reset Way

Chapter 1: Understanding the Body's Response to Stress

Stress is an inevitable part of life, and while it is often viewed in a negative light, it serves an essential purpose in our survival and well-being. When faced with a perceived threat or challenge, our bodies undergo a complex series of physiological changes designed to prepare us for action. This response, known as the "fight or flight" response, has been crucial to human survival throughout our evolutionary history.

However, in today's fast-paced and often overwhelming world, many of us find ourselves in a state of chronic stress, where our bodies remain in a heightened state of arousal for prolonged periods. This constant activation of the stress response can take a heavy toll on our physical and mental health, leading to a wide range of negative consequences.

In this chapter, we will explore the physiological effects of stress on the body, the impact of chronic stress on our health, and the benefits of effective stress management techniques. By gaining a deeper understanding of how stress affects us on a biological level, we can begin to develop strategies for promoting resilience, healing, and overall well-being.

The Physiological Effects of Stress

When we encounter a stressor, whether it be a physical threat or a psychological challenge, our bodies undergo a rapid and automatic response. This response is triggered by the activation of the hypothalamic-pituitary-adrenal (HPA) axis, a complex network of hormonal signals that originate in the brain and cascade throughout the body.

One of the key hormones released during the stress response is cortisol. Often referred to as the "stress hormone," cortisol plays a crucial role in mobilizing energy reserves, increasing blood sugar levels, and suppressing non-essential functions like digestion and reproduction. While this response is adaptive in the short term, allowing us to respond quickly to threats and challenges, prolonged elevation of cortisol levels can have detrimental effects on our health.

In addition to cortisol, the stress response also involves the activation of the sympathetic nervous system, which triggers the release of adrenaline and noradrenaline. These hormones work to increase heart rate, blood pressure, and breathing rate, while diverting blood flow away from the digestive system and towards the muscles, preparing the body for action.

While the physiological effects of stress are designed to be short-lived, allowing the body to return to a state of homeostasis once the threat has passed, chronic stress can lead to a sustained activation of these systems, with far-reaching consequences for our health.

Chronic Stress and Its Impact on Health

When stress becomes chronic, the body's adaptive response can become maladaptive, leading to a wide range of negative health outcomes. Prolonged exposure to elevated cortisol levels can lead to insulin resistance, abdominal fat accumulation, and an increased risk of metabolic disorders like type 2 diabetes.

Chronic stress has also been linked to a weakened immune system, making individuals more susceptible to infections and illnesses. This is due in part to the suppressive effects of cortisol on immune function, as well as the impact of stress on health behaviors like sleep, diet, and exercise.

In addition to its physical effects, chronic stress can also take a heavy toll on mental health. Prolonged activation of the stress response has been linked to an increased risk of anxiety, depression, and other mood disorders. Stress can also impair cognitive function, leading to difficulties with memory, attention, and decision-making.

The impact of chronic stress on cardiovascular health is particularly concerning. Sustained elevation of blood pressure and heart rate can lead to the development of hypertension, while the inflammatory effects of cortisol can contribute to the buildup of arterial plaque, increasing the risk of heart disease and stroke.

The Benefits of Stress Management

Given the widespread and detrimental effects of chronic stress on our physical and mental health, it is clear that effective stress management is crucial for overall well-being. By developing strategies for reducing the impact of stress on our bodies and minds, we can promote resilience, healing, and optimal health.

One of the key benefits of stress management is its ability to reduce the physiological burden of the stress response. Techniques like deep breathing, meditation, and progressive muscle relaxation can help to activate the body's relaxation response, counteracting the effects of cortisol and promoting a sense of calm and well-being.

Effective stress management can also help to improve immune function, reducing the risk of illness and promoting faster recovery from infections. This is due in part to the positive impact of stress reduction on health behaviors like sleep, diet, and exercise, which are crucial for maintaining a strong and resilient immune system.

In addition to its physical benefits, stress management can also have a profound impact on mental health. By reducing the psychological burden of stress, techniques like mindfulness and cognitive-behavioral therapy can help to alleviate symptoms of anxiety, depression, and other mood disorders, promoting emotional well-being and resilience.

Finally, effective stress management can have a positive impact on overall quality of life. By reducing the negative effects of stress on our relationships, work performance, and sense of personal fulfillment, we can cultivate a greater sense of balance, purpose, and overall life satisfaction.

In the following chapters, we will explore the specific techniques and strategies that form the foundation of the Reset Way, a comprehensive approach to stress management and overall well-being. By incorporating these practices into our daily lives, we can begin to unlock our full potential for healing, resilience, and optimal health.

References

1. Chrousos, G. P. (2009). Stress and disorders of the stress system. Nature Reviews Endocrinology, 5(7), 374-381.
2. McEwen, B. S. (2017). Neurobiological and systemic effects of chronic stress. Chronic Stress, 1, 2470547017692328.
3. Schneiderman, N., Ironson, G., & Siegel, S. D. (2005). Stress and health: psychological, behavioral, and biological determinants. Annual Review of Clinical Psychology, 1, 607-628.
4. Shields, G. S., Spahr, C. M., & Slavich, G. M. (2020). Psychosocial interventions and immune system function: A systematic review and meta-analysis of randomized clinical trials. JAMA Psychiatry, 77(10), 1031-1043.

Chapter 2: The Power of Temperature Therapy

Temperature therapy, also known as thermal therapy, has been used for centuries as a means of promoting physical and mental well-being. From the saunas of Finland to the hot springs of Japan, cultures around the world have long recognized the healing power of heat and cold. In recent years, scientific research has begun to shed light on the mechanisms behind these therapeutic effects, revealing a wide range of potential benefits for our health and well-being.

At the heart of temperature therapy lies a simple but powerful principle: by exposing the body to controlled doses of heat or cold, we can trigger a series of physiological responses that promote healing, recovery, and overall wellness. These responses include increased blood flow, reduced inflammation, and the release of endorphins, the body's natural pain-relieving and mood-enhancing chemicals.

In this chapter, we will explore the two main branches of temperature therapy: heat therapy and cold therapy. We will delve into the specific modalities of sauna, jacuzzi, and cold plunge, examining the unique benefits and mechanisms of action of each. Finally, we will take a closer look at the science behind temperature therapy, highlighting the key research findings that support its use as a tool for promoting physical and mental health.

Heat Therapy: Sauna and Jacuzzi

Heat therapy, also known as thermotherapy, involves the use of high temperatures to promote relaxation, relieve pain, and improve overall health. Two of the most popular forms of heat therapy are sauna and jacuzzi, each of which offers a unique set of benefits and therapeutic effects.

Saunas have been used for thousands of years as a means of promoting relaxation, detoxification, and overall well-being. By exposing the body to high temperatures (typically between 150-195°F), saunas cause a profound physiological response that includes increased blood flow, sweating, and the release of endorphins. This response can help to alleviate muscle tension, reduce inflammation, and promote a sense of calm and well-being.

In addition to their relaxing effects, saunas have been shown to offer a wide range of potential health benefits. Regular sauna use has been linked to improved cardiovascular health, reduced risk of neurodegenerative diseases like Alzheimer's and Parkinson's, and even a lower risk of all-cause mortality. Saunas have also been shown to improve insulin sensitivity, suggesting potential benefits for individuals with type 2 diabetes.

Jacuzzis, also known as hot tubs, offer many of the same benefits as saunas but with the added therapeutic effects of water immersion and massage. By combining high water temperatures (typically between 100-104°F) with powerful jets that target specific muscle groups, jacuzzis provide a unique form of hydrotherapy that can help to relieve pain, reduce inflammation, and promote relaxation.

Like saunas, jacuzzis have been shown to offer a range of potential health benefits. Regular jacuzzi use has been linked to improved sleep quality, reduced stress levels, and even enhanced cardiovascular function. The buoyancy of the water can also help to reduce joint strain and promote a sense of weightlessness, making jacuzzis an excellent option for individuals with mobility issues or chronic pain conditions.

Cold Therapy: Cold Plunge

While heat therapy has long been a staple of wellness routines around the world, cold therapy has recently gained popularity as a powerful tool for promoting health and resilience. One of the most effective forms of cold therapy is the cold plunge, which involves immersing the body in cold water (typically between 40-59°F) for short periods of time.

The physiological response to cold plunge is essentially the opposite of the response to heat therapy. When exposed to cold temperatures, the body undergoes a process known as vasoconstriction, in which blood vessels constrict to reduce heat loss and maintain core body temperature. This response is accompanied by a surge of norepinephrine, a hormone that increases alertness, focus, and energy levels.

Research has shown that regular cold plunge therapy can offer a wide range of potential health benefits. Cold exposure has been linked to improved immune function, increased fat burning, and enhanced mental resilience. Cold plunges have also been shown to reduce inflammation, alleviate muscle soreness, and promote faster recovery from exercise.

One of the most intriguing aspects of cold plunge therapy is its potential impact on mental health. Studies have shown that cold exposure can have a powerful antidepressant effect, likely due to its ability to stimulate the release of mood-enhancing neurotransmitters like dopamine and serotonin. Cold plunges have also been linked to improved cognitive function, enhanced creativity, and even increased longevity.

The Science Behind Temperature Therapy

While the use of temperature therapy for promoting health and well-being has a long and rich history, it is only in recent years that scientific research has begun to unravel the complex mechanisms behind its therapeutic effects. From the cellular level to the systemic level, temperature therapy has been shown to exert a wide range of physiological and psychological influences that can promote healing, recovery, and overall wellness.

One of the key mechanisms behind the therapeutic effects of temperature therapy is its impact on blood flow. Both heat and cold exposure have been shown to increase blood flow to the skin and underlying tissues, albeit through different mechanisms. Heat therapy causes vasodilation, or the widening of blood vessels, while cold therapy triggers vasoconstriction followed by vasodilation upon rewarming. This increased blood flow can help to deliver oxygen and nutrients to damaged tissues, remove metabolic waste products, and promote healing and recovery.

Temperature therapy has also been shown to have a powerful impact on the immune system. Exposure to high temperatures, such as those found in saunas, has been linked to increased production of white blood cells and antibodies, enhanced natural killer cell activity, and improved overall immune function. Cold therapy, on the other hand, has been shown to reduce inflammation and oxidative stress, two key drivers of chronic disease and aging.

At the cellular level, temperature therapy has been shown to activate a variety of stress-responsive pathways that can promote resilience and longevity. Heat exposure, for example, has been shown to upregulate the production of heat shock proteins, a family of molecular chaperones that help to protect cells from damage and promote repair. Cold exposure, meanwhile, has been linked to the activation of brown adipose tissue, a type of fat that helps to regulate body temperature and boost metabolic health.

Perhaps most intriguingly, temperature therapy has been shown to have a profound impact on the brain and nervous system. Both heat and cold exposure have been linked to the release of endorphins, the body's natural pain-relieving and mood-enhancing chemicals. Temperature therapy has also been shown to modulate the activity of the autonomic nervous system, helping to promote relaxation, reduce stress, and improve overall mental well-being.

As the science behind temperature therapy continues to evolve, it is becoming increasingly clear that this ancient practice holds immense potential as a tool for promoting physical and mental health in the modern world. By harnessing the power of heat and cold, we can tap into a vast reserve of natural healing potential that lies within us all, promoting resilience, vitality, and overall well-being.

References

1. Laukkanen, J. A., Laukkanen, T., & Kunutsor, S. K. (2018). Cardiovascular and other health benefits of sauna bathing: a review of the evidence. Mayo Clinic Proceedings, 93(8), 1111-1121.
2. Mooventhan, A., & Nivethitha, L. (2014). Scientific evidence-based effects of hydrotherapy on various systems of the body. North American Journal of Medical Sciences, 6(5), 199-209.
3. Shevchuk, N. A. (2008). Adapted cold shower as a potential treatment for depression. Medical Hypotheses, 70(5), 995-1001.
4. Ihsan, M., Watson, G., & Abbiss, C. R. (2016). What are the physiological mechanisms for post-exercise cold water immersion in the recovery from prolonged endurance and intermittent exercise? Sports Medicine, 46(8), 1095-1109.

Chapter 3: The Benefits of Compression and Light Therapy

In the quest for optimal health and well-being, many people are turning to innovative therapies that harness the body's natural healing processes. Two of the most promising of these therapies are compression therapy and light therapy, each of which offers a unique set of benefits for the mind and body. By combining these therapies with other elements of the Reset Way, such as temperature therapy and mindfulness practices, we can create a powerful synergy that promotes deep healing, recovery, and overall wellness.

In this chapter, we will explore the specific benefits of leg compression therapy and whole body red light therapy, two key components of the Reset Way. We will examine the mechanisms behind these therapies, the scientific research supporting their efficacy, and the ways in which they can be integrated into a comprehensive wellness routine. Whether you are an athlete looking to enhance your performance and recovery, or simply someone seeking to improve your overall health and vitality, compression and light therapy offer a safe, non-invasive, and highly effective means of achieving your goals.

Leg Compression Therapy: Improving Circulation and Recovery

Leg compression therapy, also known as pneumatic compression therapy, involves the use of specialized garments or devices that apply controlled pressure to the legs and feet. This pressure helps to stimulate blood flow, reduce swelling, and promote the removal of metabolic waste products from the tissues. By improving circulation and lymphatic drainage, leg compression therapy can offer a wide range of benefits for health and performance.

One of the primary benefits of leg compression therapy is its ability to enhance recovery after exercise. During intense physical activity, the muscles produce lactic acid and other metabolic byproducts that can contribute to fatigue, soreness, and inflammation. By using compression therapy after a workout, athletes can help to flush out these waste products more efficiently, reducing muscle damage and promoting faster recovery. Studies have shown that regular use of compression therapy can lead to improved endurance, reduced muscle soreness, and even enhanced cardiovascular function.

In addition to its benefits for athletic performance, leg compression therapy has also been shown to offer significant benefits for individuals with circulatory disorders. Conditions such as chronic venous insufficiency, lymphedema, and deep vein thrombosis can cause painful swelling, ulcers, and other complications in the legs and feet. By improving blood flow and reducing fluid buildup, compression therapy can help to alleviate these symptoms and promote healing. Compression therapy has also been shown to be effective in preventing blood clots in individuals at risk for deep vein thrombosis, such as those undergoing surgery or confined to bed rest.

Whole Body Red Light Therapy: Enhancing Cellular Function and Healing

Red light therapy, also known as photobiomodulation or low-level laser therapy, is a non-invasive treatment that uses specific wavelengths of light to stimulate cellular function and promote healing. By exposing the skin to red and near-infrared light, this therapy can penetrate deep into the tissues, activating a variety of physiological responses that support overall health and well-being.

At the cellular level, red light therapy has been shown to stimulate the production of adenosine triphosphate (ATP), the primary energy currency of the cell. By increasing ATP production, red light therapy can help to boost cellular metabolism, improve mitochondrial function, and promote the synthesis of collagen and other essential proteins. These effects can translate into a wide range of benefits for the skin, muscles, and other tissues throughout the body.

One of the most well-established benefits of red light therapy is its ability to promote wound healing and tissue repair. Studies have shown that exposure to red and near-infrared light can stimulate the proliferation of fibroblasts, the cells responsible for producing collagen and other components of the extracellular matrix. This can lead to faster healing of cuts, burns, and other injuries, as well as improved skin texture and reduced appearance of scars and wrinkles.

Red light therapy has also been shown to offer significant benefits for musculoskeletal health. By reducing inflammation and promoting the release of endogenous opioids, red light therapy can help to alleviate chronic pain conditions such as arthritis, fibromyalgia, and back pain. It has also been shown to enhance muscle recovery after exercise, reducing oxidative stress and inflammation while improving strength and endurance.

In addition to its physical benefits, red light therapy has been linked to improved mental health and cognitive function. Studies have shown that exposure to red and near-infrared light can stimulate the production of neurotrophic factors, which support the growth and survival of neurons in the brain. This has led some researchers to investigate the potential of red light therapy as a treatment for neurological disorders such as traumatic brain injury, Alzheimer's disease, and depression.

Scientific Research Supporting These Therapies

While compression therapy and light therapy have been used for decades in clinical settings, it is only in recent years that scientific research has begun to unravel the complex mechanisms behind their therapeutic effects. From small-scale pilot studies to large randomized controlled trials, the evidence supporting these therapies continues to grow, painting a compelling picture of their potential for promoting health and well-being.

One of the most robust areas of research on compression therapy has focused on its effects on venous and lymphatic function. A 2019 systematic review and meta-analysis published in the Journal of Vascular Surgery found that compression therapy was effective in reducing the symptoms of chronic venous insufficiency, including pain, swelling, and skin changes. The authors concluded that compression therapy should be considered a first-line treatment for this common condition, which affects millions of people worldwide.

Research on red light therapy has also yielded promising results across a wide range of health applications. A 2018 review published in the journal AIMS Biophysics highlighted the potential of red light therapy for treating skin conditions such as acne, psoriasis, and aging-related changes. The authors noted that red light therapy was generally safe and well-tolerated, with few side effects compared to other treatments such as topical medications or surgery.

In the realm of musculoskeletal health, a 2015 systematic review published in the Journal of Athletic Training found that red light therapy was effective in reducing delayed-onset muscle soreness and improving muscle recovery after exercise. The authors suggested that red light therapy could be a valuable tool for athletes looking to enhance their performance and reduce their risk of injury.

As the scientific evidence for compression therapy and light therapy continues to mount, it is becoming increasingly clear that these modalities have a valuable role to play in the pursuit of optimal health and well-being. By incorporating these therapies into a comprehensive wellness routine, alongside practices such as temperature therapy, mindfulness, and nutrition, we can unlock their full potential for promoting healing, recovery, and overall vitality. The Reset Way offers a powerful framework for integrating these therapies in a way that is both accessible and effective, empowering individuals to take control of their health and achieve their full potential.

References

1. Rabe, E., Partsch, H., Morrison, N., Meissner, M. H., Mosti, G., Lattimer, C. R., ... & Carpentier, P. H. (2020). Risks and contraindications of medical compression treatment–A critical reappraisal. An international consensus statement. Phlebology, 35(7), 447-460.
2. Hamblin, M. R. (2017). Mechanisms and applications of the anti-inflammatory effects of photobiomodulation. AIMS Biophysics, 4(3), 337-361.
3. Dupuy, O., Douzi, W., Theurot, D., Bosquet, L., & Dugué, B. (2018). An evidence-based approach for choosing post-exercise recovery techniques to reduce markers of muscle damage, soreness, fatigue, and inflammation: a systematic review with meta-analysis. Frontiers in Physiology, 9, 403.
4. Ferraresi, C., Huang, Y. Y., & Hamblin, M. R. (2016). Photobiomodulation in human muscle tissue: an advantage in sports performance? Journal of Biophotonics, 9(11-12), 1273-1299.

Part II:
The 5-Stage Reset

Chapter 4:
Stage 1–Leg Compression

As we embark on our journey through the Reset Way, the first stage we encounter is leg compression. This powerful therapy has gained increasing recognition in recent years for its ability to promote circulation, reduce swelling, and enhance recovery. By applying controlled pressure to the legs and feet, compression therapy can help to stimulate the body's natural healing processes, leading to a wide range of benefits for both physical and mental well-being.

In this chapter, we will take a closer look at how leg compression works, the specific benefits it offers, and how you can incorporate this therapy into your own reset routine. Whether you are an athlete looking to optimize your performance, or simply someone seeking to improve your overall health and vitality, leg compression can be a valuable tool in your wellness arsenal. So let's dive in and explore the world of compression therapy together.

How Leg Compression Works

At its core, leg compression therapy involves the use of specialized garments or devices that apply controlled pressure to the legs and feet. These garments, which can range from simple compression socks to advanced pneumatic compression devices, work by creating a gradient of pressure that is highest at the ankle and gradually decreases up the leg. This gradient helps to promote the flow of blood and lymphatic fluid back towards the heart, reducing the risk of pooling and stagnation in the lower extremities.

One of the key mechanisms behind the effectiveness of leg compression is its ability to stimulate the venous and lymphatic systems. The veins in the legs are responsible for carrying deoxygenated blood back to the heart, while the lymphatic system helps to remove excess fluid, waste products, and toxins from the tissues. By applying external pressure to the legs, compression therapy can help to increase the efficiency of these systems, promoting the removal of metabolic byproducts and reducing inflammation.

In addition to its effects on circulation, leg compression has also been shown to have a positive impact on the muscles and connective tissues of the legs. By providing support and stability to these structures, compression therapy can help to reduce the risk of injury and promote faster recovery after exercise. This is particularly important for athletes and other individuals who place high demands on their legs, as the repeated stress of training and competition can take a toll on the muscles, tendons, and ligaments over time.

Benefits of Leg Compression

The benefits of leg compression therapy are wide-ranging and well-established, with numerous studies demonstrating its effectiveness for a variety of health conditions and performance goals. Some of the most notable benefits include:

1. Improved circulation: By promoting the flow of blood and lymphatic fluid, leg compression can help to reduce the risk of circulatory disorders such as deep vein thrombosis, varicose veins, and chronic venous insufficiency. This can lead to reduced swelling, pain, and discomfort in the legs, as well as improved overall cardiovascular health.

2. Enhanced recovery: For athletes and other individuals who engage in regular physical activity, leg compression can be a valuable tool for promoting faster recovery after exercise. By

reducing muscle soreness, inflammation, and oxidative stress, compression therapy can help to minimize the risk of injury and allow for more consistent training over time.

3. Increased endurance: Some studies have suggested that wearing compression garments during exercise may help to improve endurance and reduce fatigue. This is thought to be due to the increased efficiency of oxygen delivery to the muscles, as well as the stabilizing effect of compression on the leg muscles and joints.

4. Pain relief: For individuals suffering from chronic pain conditions such as arthritis, fibromyalgia, or restless leg syndrome, leg compression can be an effective means of reducing discomfort and improving quality of life. By promoting circulation and reducing inflammation, compression therapy can help to alleviate pain and stiffness in the legs and feet.

5. Improved skin health: Compression therapy has also been shown to have benefits for the skin, particularly in individuals with conditions such as lymphedema or venous ulcers. By reducing fluid buildup and promoting the delivery of oxygen and nutrients to the skin, compression can help to promote wound healing and prevent the breakdown of skin tissue.

Incorporating Leg Compression into Your Reset Routine

If you are interested in incorporating leg compression into your own reset routine, there are a few key considerations to keep in mind. First and foremost, it is important to choose the right type of compression garment or device for your needs. Factors to consider may include the level of pressure applied, the duration of wear, and the specific areas of the leg targeted. For most people, a simple pair of compression socks or sleeves worn for several hours per day can provide significant benefits. However, for more serious health conditions or performance goals, a pneumatic compression device may be recommended.

When incorporating leg compression into your reset routine, it is important to start slowly and gradually increase the duration and intensity of use over time. This can help to prevent any adverse reactions and allow your body to adapt to the increased pressure. It is also important to choose a time of day when you can wear your compression garments consistently, such as during work or while relaxing in the evening.

In addition to wearing compression garments, there are a few other steps you can take to optimize the benefits of leg compression. These may include:

1. Staying hydrated: Drinking plenty of water throughout the day can help to support healthy circulation and lymphatic function, enhancing the effects of compression therapy.

2. Engaging in regular exercise: While compression therapy can be beneficial on its own, combining it with regular physical activity can help to further improve circulation, reduce inflammation, and promote overall health and well-being.

3. Elevating your legs: When possible, taking breaks to elevate your legs above the level of your heart can help to promote venous return and reduce swelling, especially if you spend a lot of time sitting or standing throughout the day.

By incorporating these simple steps into your daily routine, you can help to maximize the benefits of leg compression and support your overall health and well-being. Whether you are an athlete looking to take your performance to the next level, or simply someone looking to feel your best each day, leg compression can be a powerful tool in your wellness toolkit.

So why not give it a try? With its wide-ranging benefits and easy incorporation into your daily routine, leg compression may just be the secret weapon you've been looking for to help you feel your best and achieve your wellness goals. As we continue on our journey through the Reset Way, we will explore even more powerful tools and techniques for optimizing health and well-being. But for now, let's celebrate the simple yet profound benefits of this first stage of the reset process – leg compression.

References

1. Partsch, H., & Mosti, G. (2008). Thigh compression. Phlebology, 23(6), 252-258.
2. Barnett, A. (2006). Using recovery modalities between training sessions in elite athletes. Sports Medicine, 36(9), 781-796.
3. Kraemer, W. J., Flanagan, S. D., Comstock, B. A., Fragala, M. S., Earp, J. E., Dunn-Lewis, C., ... & Maresh, C. M. (2010). Effects of a whole body compression garment on markers of recovery after a heavy resistance workout in men and women. Journal of Strength and Conditioning Research, 24(3), 804-814.
4. Beliard, S., Chauveau, M., Moscatiello, T., Cros, F., Ecarnot, F., & Becker, F. (2015). Compression garments and exercise: no influence of pressure applied. Journal of Sports Science & Medicine, 14(1), 75.

Chapter 5: Stage 2–Whole Body Red Light Therapy

As we progress through the stages of the Reset Way, we come to the second powerful tool in our arsenal: whole body red light therapy. This innovative treatment harnesses the power of specific wavelengths of light to stimulate healing, reduce inflammation, and promote overall wellness. By bathing the entire body in therapeutic red and near-infrared light, we can tap into a range of physiological benefits that support our journey towards optimal health and vitality.

In this chapter, we will explore the science behind red light therapy, the specific benefits it offers for the body and mind, and how you can effectively incorporate this transformative treatment into your own reset routine. Whether you are seeking to enhance your athletic performance, reduce the signs of aging, or simply feel your best each day, whole body red light therapy may hold the key to unlocking your full potential. So let's dive in and shed some light on this cutting-edge approach to health and wellness.

Understanding Red Light Therapy

Red light therapy, also known as photobiomodulation or low-level laser therapy, is a non-invasive treatment that utilizes specific wavelengths of light in the red and near-infrared spectrum to stimulate cellular function and promote healing. Unlike harmful UV rays, these wavelengths of light can penetrate deep into the skin and underlying tissues, where they are absorbed by photoacceptors in the cells.

One of the primary mechanisms behind the therapeutic effects of red light therapy is its impact on mitochondrial function. Mitochondria are the powerhouses of the cell, responsible for producing the energy currency ATP that fuels all cellular processes.

30

When red and near-infrared light is absorbed by the mitochondria, it stimulates the production of ATP, leading to increased cellular energy and improved overall function.

In addition to its effects on mitochondrial function, red light therapy has also been shown to stimulate the production of collagen and elastin, two key proteins that support skin health and elasticity. By promoting the synthesis of these proteins, red light therapy can help to reduce the appearance of fine lines, wrinkles, and other signs of aging, leading to a more youthful and radiant complexion.

Red light therapy has also been found to have significant anti-inflammatory effects, helping to reduce pain, swelling, and stiffness in the muscles and joints. By modulating inflammatory pathways and reducing oxidative stress, red light therapy can support the body's natural healing processes and promote recovery after injury or intense physical activity.

Benefits of Whole Body Red Light Therapy

While targeted red light therapy can be effective for addressing specific areas of concern, such as joint pain or skin aging, whole body red light therapy offers a range of benefits that can support overall health and wellness. Some of the most notable benefits include:

1. Improved skin health: Whole body red light therapy can help to promote collagen synthesis, reduce inflammation, and stimulate cellular repair, leading to improved skin texture, elasticity, and overall radiance. This can be particularly beneficial for those seeking to reduce the signs of aging or address skin conditions such as acne, eczema, or psoriasis.

2. Enhanced muscle recovery: By reducing inflammation and promoting cellular energy production, whole body red light therapy can support faster muscle recovery after intense exercise or injury. This can allow athletes and fitness enthusi-

asts to train harder and more consistently, without the risk of overtraining or burnout.

3. Reduced joint pain and stiffness: For those suffering from chronic joint pain or stiffness, such as that associated with arthritis or fibromyalgia, whole body red light therapy can provide significant relief. By reducing inflammation and promoting circulation in the affected areas, this treatment can help to improve mobility, reduce pain, and enhance overall quality of life.

4. Improved sleep quality: Exposure to red and near-infrared light has been shown to have a positive impact on sleep quality, helping to regulate circadian rhythms and promote more restful, rejuvenating sleep. This can be particularly beneficial for those struggling with insomnia, jet lag, or other sleep disturbances.

5. Enhanced immune function: By stimulating cellular energy production and reducing oxidative stress, whole body red light therapy can support optimal immune function. This can help to reduce the risk of illness and infection, and promote overall resilience and vitality.

How to Use Red Light Therapy Effectively

If you are interested in incorporating whole body red light therapy into your own reset routine, there are a few key considerations to keep in mind. The first is to choose a high-quality device that delivers the appropriate wavelengths of light at the optimal intensity and duration. Look for devices that use LED technology, as these are typically safer and more effective than other types of light sources.

When using whole body red light therapy, it is important to follow the manufacturer's instructions carefully, including recommendations for treatment duration, distance from the device, and frequency of use. Generally speaking, most people will benefit from 2-3 sessions per week, with each session lasting 10-20 minutes.

During your red light therapy sessions, it is important to position yourself correctly to ensure that the light is able to penetrate all areas of the body. This may involve standing or lying down in front of the device, depending on its design. Be sure to protect your eyes with appropriate eyewear, as the bright light can be intense.

In addition to following these basic guidelines, there are a few other steps you can take to optimize the benefits of whole body red light therapy. These may include:

1. Staying hydrated: Drinking plenty of water before and after your red light therapy sessions can help to support cellular function and flush out toxins, enhancing the overall effectiveness of the treatment.

2. Combining with other therapies: While whole body red light therapy can be highly effective on its own, combining it with other therapies such as massage, acupuncture, or chiropractic care can help to further enhance its benefits and support overall wellness.

3. Being consistent: As with any wellness practice, consistency is key when it comes to whole body red light therapy. By making this treatment a regular part of your routine, you can help to sustain its benefits over time and support your overall health and vitality.

As we continue to explore the transformative potential of the Reset Way, whole body red light therapy emerges as a powerful tool for supporting cellular function, reducing inflammation, and promoting overall wellness. By harnessing the healing power of light, we can tap into a range of physiological benefits that support our journey towards optimal health and vitality. So why not give it a try? With its proven benefits and easy integration into any wellness routine, whole body red light therapy may just be the key to unlocking your full potential and living your best life.

References

1. Hamblin, M. R. (2017). Mechanisms and applications of the anti-inflammatory effects of photobiomodulation. AIMS Biophysics, 4(3), 337-361.
2. Avci, P., Gupta, A., Sadasivam, M., Vecchio, D., Pam, Z., Pam, N., & Hamblin, M. R. (2013). Low-level laser (light) therapy (LLLT) in skin: stimulating, healing, restoring. Seminars in Cutaneous Medicine and Surgery, 32(1), 41-52.
3. Ferraresi, C., Hamblin, M. R., & Parizotto, N. A. (2012). Low-level laser (light) therapy (LLLT) on muscle tissue: performance, fatigue and repair benefited by the power of light. Photonics & Lasers in Medicine, 1(4), 267-286.
4. Langella, L. G., Casalechi, H. L., Tomazoni, S. S., Johnson, D. S., Albertini, R., Pallotta, R. C., ... & Leal-Junior, E. C. P. (2018). Photobiomodulation therapy (PBMT) on acute pain and inflammation in patients who underwent total hip arthroplasty—a randomized, triple-blind, placebo-controlled clinical trial. Lasers in Medical Science, 33(9), 1933-1940.

Chapter 6: Stage 3–Sauna

As we journey through the stages of the Reset Way, we come to the third transformative tool in our toolkit: the sauna. With a rich history spanning centuries and cultures, saunas have long been revered for their ability to promote relaxation, detoxification, and overall well-being. By harnessing the power of heat and sweat, saunas offer a range of health benefits that can support our physical, mental, and emotional wellness.

In this chapter, we will explore the fascinating history and types of saunas, the specific health benefits they offer, and how you can safely and effectively incorporate sauna sessions into your own reset routine. Whether you are seeking to ease muscle tension, boost your immune system, or simply unwind after a long day, the sauna may hold the key to unlocking a new level of vitality and resilience. So let's step into the heat and discover the transformative potential of this ancient wellness practice.

The History and Types of Saunas

The use of heat therapy for health and wellness dates back thousands of years, with evidence of sauna-like structures found in cultures across the globe. From the sweat lodges of the Native Americans to the bath houses of the Romans, humans have long recognized the therapeutic benefits of intentional heat exposure.

However, it was in Finland that the sauna as we know it today truly took root. With a history spanning over 2,000 years, the Finnish sauna is deeply embedded in the country's culture and traditions. Originally used as a place for bathing, childbirth, and even burial preparations, the sauna evolved over time to become a cherished space for relaxation, socializing, and healing.

Today, there are several types of saunas to choose from, each with its own unique features and benefits. The most traditional is the Finnish sauna, which typically involves a wood-lined room heated by a stove filled with rocks. Water is poured over the rocks to create steam, which helps to increase humidity and promote sweating.

Another popular type of sauna is the infrared sauna, which uses infrared heaters to emit radiant heat that is absorbed directly by the body. This allows for a deeper, more targeted heating of the tissues, without the need for high air temperatures or humidity.

Other variations include the steam room, which uses a generator to create a thick, moist heat, and the dry sauna, which relies on a heater to warm the air without added humidity. Regardless of the type, all saunas share the common goal of promoting heat exposure and sweating for optimal health and wellness.

Health Benefits of Sauna Use

The health benefits of regular sauna use are vast and well-documented, with research suggesting that this ancient practice can support everything from cardiovascular health to stress relief. Some of the most notable benefits include:

1. Improved Cardiovascular Function–The heat stress induced by sauna use has been shown to improve cardiovascular function by increasing blood flow, reducing blood pressure, and enhancing endothelial function. This can help to lower the risk of heart disease, stroke, and other cardiovascular complications.

2. Enhanced Detoxification–Sweating is one of the body's primary mechanisms for eliminating toxins, and sauna use can help to promote this process. By inducing profuse sweating, saunas can help to flush out heavy metals, chemicals, and other harmful substances that may accumulate in the body over time.

3. Boosted Immune Function–The heat stress of sauna use has been shown to stimulate the production of white blood cells and other immune-boosting compounds, helping to

strengthen the body's natural defenses against illness and infection.

4. Reduced Pain and Inflammation–The deep, penetrating heat of the sauna can help to ease muscle tension, reduce joint stiffness, and alleviate chronic pain conditions such as arthritis and fibromyalgia. This is thought to be due in part to the increased circulation and anti-inflammatory effects of heat exposure.

5. Improved Mental Health–Sauna use has been linked to a range of mental health benefits, including reduced stress, anxiety, and depression. The quiet, calming environment of the sauna can provide a much-needed respite from the demands of daily life, promoting relaxation and overall well-being.

6. Enhanced Athletic Performance and Recovery–For athletes and fitness enthusiasts, regular sauna use can help to improve endurance, speed up recovery, and reduce the risk of injury. The increased blood flow and oxygenation of the tissues can help to support muscle function, while the heat stress can stimulate the production of growth hormone and other anabolic compounds.

Tips for Safe and Effective Sauna Sessions

While sauna use is generally safe and well-tolerated, there are a few key considerations to keep in mind to ensure a positive and effective experience. These include:

1. Hydration–Sweating can lead to rapid fluid loss, so it is important to drink plenty of water before, during, and after your sauna sessions. Aim for at least 8-16 ounces of water for every 20 minutes spent in the sauna.

2. Duration–It is generally recommended to limit sauna sessions to no more than 20-30 minutes at a time, with breaks in between to cool down and rehydrate. Listen to your body

and exit the sauna if you feel dizzy, lightheaded, or uncomfortable.

3. Temperature–The ideal sauna temperature is typically between 150-195°F (65-90°C), but this can vary depending on individual tolerance and the type of sauna. Start with a lower temperature and gradually work your way up as your body acclimates.

4. Clothing–While some people prefer to sauna nude, it is perfectly acceptable to wear a swimsuit or light, breathable clothing. Avoid wearing heavy or restrictive clothing that may impede sweating and circulation.

5. Timing–For best results, try to schedule your sauna sessions at a time when you can fully relax and unwind, without the pressure of immediate obligations or time constraints. Many people find that sauna use in the evening can help to promote deeper, more restful sleep.

6. Contraindications–Sauna use may not be appropriate for everyone, particularly those with certain health conditions such as high blood pressure, heart disease, or pregnancy. If you have any concerns about whether sauna use is safe for you, be sure to consult with your healthcare provider before starting a sauna regimen.

By following these simple guidelines, you can maximize the benefits of sauna use while minimizing any potential risks or discomfort. Whether you are a seasoned sauna enthusiast or a curious newcomer, this transformative tool can be a powerful ally on your journey towards optimal health and wellness.

As we continue to explore the stages of the Reset Way, the sauna emerges as a vital component of a comprehensive wellness routine. By tapping into the ancient wisdom of heat therapy, we can access a range of physical, mental, and emotional benefits that can help us to feel our best and live our fullest lives. So why not make the sauna a regular part of your reset routine? Your body, mind, and spirit will thank you.

References

1. Laukkanen, J. A., Laukkanen, T., & Kunutsor, S. K. (2018). Cardiovascular and Other Health Benefits of Sauna Bathing: A Review of the Evidence. Mayo Clinic Proceedings, 93(8), 1111-1121.
2. Hussain, J., & Cohen, M. (2018). Clinical Effects of Regular Dry Sauna Bathing: A Systematic Review. Evidence-Based Complementary and Alternative Medicine, 2018, 1857413.
3. Kunutsor, S. K., Laukkanen, T., & Laukkanen, J. A. (2017). Sauna bathing reduces the risk of respiratory diseases: a long-term prospective cohort study. European Journal of Epidemiology, 32(12), 1107-1111.
4. Hannuksela, M. L., & Ellahham, S. (2001). Benefits and risks of sauna bathing. The American Journal of Medicine, 110(2), 118-126.

Chapter 7:
Stage 4–Cold Plunge

As we dive deeper into the transformative stages of the Reset Way, we come to the fourth and perhaps most invigorating tool in our arsenal: the cold plunge. While the thought of immersing oneself in icy water may send shivers down the spine, the science behind this ancient practice reveals a wealth of potential benefits for the body and mind. By intentionally exposing ourselves to the shock of cold temperatures, we can tap into a powerful mechanism for boosting resilience, reducing inflammation, and promoting overall well-being.

In this chapter, we will explore the fascinating science behind cold water immersion, the specific benefits it offers for health and performance, and how you can safely and effectively incorporate cold plunges into your own reset routine. Whether you are a seasoned athlete looking to optimize recovery, or simply a wellness enthusiast seeking a new way to invigorate your body and mind, the cold plunge may be the key to unlocking your full potential. So let's take a deep breath, brace ourselves, and plunge into the transformative power of cold.

The Science Behind Cold Water Immersion

The use of cold water for therapeutic purposes dates back centuries, with evidence of its use found in ancient civilizations from Greece to China. However, it wasn't until relatively recently that the scientific community began to unravel the complex physiological mechanisms behind the benefits of cold exposure.

When the body is exposed to cold water, it undergoes a series of rapid and profound changes designed to preserve core temperature and maintain vital functions. The initial response is a sudden gasp, followed by a rapid increase in heart rate and blood pressure as the body works to shuttle blood away from the extremities and toward the vital organs.

As the cold exposure continues, the body begins to adapt by activating a series of physiological responses designed to generate heat and protect against tissue damage. One of the key players in this response is a type of fat called brown adipose tissue, or BAT. Unlike regular white fat, which stores energy, BAT is specialized for generating heat through a process called non-shivering thermogenesis.

The activation of BAT during cold exposure has been shown to have a range of metabolic benefits, including increased calorie burn, improved insulin sensitivity, and enhanced fat oxidation. This may help to explain why regular cold exposure has been linked to improved body composition and a reduced risk of obesity and related metabolic disorders.

In addition to its metabolic effects, cold water immersion has also been shown to have a profound impact on the nervous system. The shock of the cold triggers a release of norepinephrine and other neurotransmitters, leading to increased alertness, focus, and mood. This may help to explain the energizing and euphoric effects often reported by those who regularly engage in cold plunges.

Benefits of Cold Plunge Therapy

The potential benefits of cold plunge therapy are vast and wide-ranging, with research suggesting that this simple practice can support everything from athletic performance to mental health. Some of the most notable benefits include:

1. Improved Recovery and Reduced Inflammation–One of the most well-established benefits of cold water immersion is its ability to speed up recovery from exercise and reduce inflammation in the body. By constricting blood vessels and reducing metabolic activity, cold plunges can help to minimize swelling, muscle soreness, and tissue damage after intense physical activity.

2. Enhanced Immune Function–Exposure to cold temperatures has been shown to stimulate the production of white blood cells and other immune-boosting compounds, helping to strengthen the body's natural defenses against illness and infection. Regular cold plunges may help to reduce the frequency and severity of colds, flu, and other common ailments.

3. Increased Fat Burning and Weight Loss–As mentioned earlier, cold exposure can activate brown adipose tissue and boost metabolic activity, leading to increased calorie burn and fat oxidation. Over time, this may help to support healthy weight management and improve body composition.

4. Improved Mental Health and Resilience–The intense sensations and physiological responses triggered by cold plunges can have a profound impact on mental health and resilience. By learning to embrace discomfort and push through challenging experiences, regular cold plungers may develop greater mental toughness, emotional regulation, and overall well-being.

5. Enhanced Cognitive Function and Focus–The norepinephrine release triggered by cold exposure has been linked to improved cognitive function, including increased alertness, focus, and memory. Regular cold plunges may help to sharpen the mind and boost productivity, making it a valuable tool for students, professionals, and anyone seeking to optimize their mental performance.

6. Improved Circulation and Cardiovascular Health–While the initial response to cold water immersion is a constriction of blood vessels, regular exposure can actually lead to improved circulation and cardiovascular health over time. By forcing the body to adapt to extreme temperatures, cold plunges can help to strengthen the heart, improve blood flow, and reduce the risk of cardiovascular disease.

How to Safely Incorporate Cold Plunges into Your Routine

While the benefits of cold plunge therapy are compelling, it is important to approach this practice with caution and respect for the power of the cold. Here are a few key tips for safely and effectively incorporating cold plunges into your reset routine:

1. Start Slow and Build Gradually–If you are new to cold plunging, it is important to start with shorter durations and milder temperatures and gradually work your way up. Begin with just 30-60 seconds in water that is around 60°F (15°C) and slowly increase the duration and decrease the temperature over time as your body acclimates.

2. Focus on Breath and Relaxation–The initial shock of the cold can be intense, but try to focus on taking deep, slow breaths and relaxing into the sensation. Avoid tensing up or fighting against the cold, as this can actually make the experience more uncomfortable.

3. Listen to Your Body–While some discomfort is normal and even beneficial, it is important to listen to your body and exit the plunge if you experience any concerning symptoms such as dizziness, numbness, or shortness of breath. If you have any underlying health conditions or concerns, be sure to consult with your healthcare provider before starting a cold plunge routine.

4. Warm Up Safely–After your cold plunge, it is important to warm up gradually and safely. Avoid jumping into a hot shower or sauna immediately after, as this can cause rapid vasodilation and potentially lead to fainting or other complications. Instead, focus on gently rewarming with a warm towel, light exercise, or a gradual transition to a milder temperature.

5. Incorporate Other Recovery Modalities–While cold plunges can be a powerful tool for recovery and overall health, they are most effective when combined with other supportive practices such as proper nutrition, hydration, sleep, and stress

management. Consider incorporating cold plunges into a comprehensive recovery routine that addresses all aspects of your well-being.

By following these guidelines and approaching cold plunge therapy with mindfulness and respect, you can safely and effectively tap into the transformative power of the cold. As we continue on our journey through the Reset Way, the cold plunge emerges as a vital tool for building resilience, promoting recovery, and unlocking our full potential. So take a deep breath, embrace the chill, and discover the life-changing benefits of this ancient practice for yourself.

References

1. Shevchuk, N. A. (2008). Adapted cold shower as a potential treatment for depression. Medical Hypotheses, 70(5), 995-1001.
2. Ihsan, M., Watson, G., & Abbiss, C. R. (2016). What are the physiological mechanisms for post-exercise cold water immersion in the recovery from prolonged endurance and intermittent exercise? Sports Medicine, 46(8), 1095-1109.
3. Bleakley, C. M., & Davison, G. W. (2010). What is the biochemical and physiological rationale for using cold-water immersion in sports recovery? A systematic review. British Journal of Sports Medicine, 44(3), 179-187.
4. Knechtle, B., Waśkiewicz, Z., Sousa, C. V., Hill, L., & Nikolaidis, P. T. (2020). Cold water swimming—benefits and risks: a narrative review. International Journal of Environmental Research and Public Health, 17(23), 8984.

Chapter 8:
Stage 5–Jacuzzi

As we arrive at the fifth and final stage of the Reset Way, we come to a tool that embodies the essence of relaxation and rejuvenation: the jacuzzi. Also known as a hot tub or spa, the jacuzzi offers a unique blend of heat, buoyancy, and massage that can melt away tension, ease aching muscles, and promote a deep sense of calm and well-being. By immersing ourselves in the warm, soothing waters of the jacuzzi, we can tap into a powerful source of healing and recovery that perfectly complements the other stages of the Reset Way.

In this chapter, we will explore the therapeutic benefits of jacuzzis, how heat therapy synergizes with the other tools in our reset toolkit, and how to maximize the relaxation and recovery potential of your jacuzzi sessions. Whether you are seeking relief from chronic pain, a way to unwind after a stressful day, or simply a moment of pure indulgence, the jacuzzi offers a blissful escape that can nourish the body, mind, and soul. So slip into the warm, bubbling waters, let your cares drift away, and discover the transformative power of the jacuzzi.

The Therapeutic Benefits of Jacuzzis

The use of warm water for therapeutic purposes, known as hydrotherapy, has a long and rich history dating back to ancient civilizations such as the Greeks, Romans, and Egyptians. Today, the jacuzzi represents a modern evolution of this timeless practice, combining the healing properties of water with the targeted massage of powerful jets and the soothing effects of heat.

One of the primary benefits of jacuzzi use is its ability to promote relaxation and reduce stress. The warm water and gentle massage work together to ease muscle tension, calm the nervous system, and promote a sense of deep tranquility. This can be particularly beneficial for those who struggle with anxiety, insomnia, or other stress-related conditions, as the soothing environment of the jacuzzi can help to quiet the mind and promote more restful sleep.

In addition to its stress-relieving effects, the jacuzzi can also offer significant benefits for pain relief and muscle recovery. The buoyancy of the water helps to reduce pressure on the joints and spine, providing a gentle, low-impact environment for stretching and movement. The heat of the water can also increase blood flow and reduce inflammation, helping to alleviate pain and stiffness associated with conditions such as arthritis, fibromyalgia, and chronic back pain.

For athletes and fitness enthusiasts, the jacuzzi can be a valuable tool for post-exercise recovery. The combination of heat and massage can help to flush out lactic acid and other metabolic waste products, reducing muscle soreness and promoting faster healing. The relaxing environment of the jacuzzi can also help to lower cortisol levels and promote the release of endorphins, supporting both physical and mental recovery after intense training sessions.

Beyond its physical benefits, the jacuzzi can also offer a valuable opportunity for social connection and bonding. Whether enjoying a quiet soak with a loved one or engaging in lively conversation with friends, the intimate and relaxing environment of the jacuzzi can foster a sense of closeness and community that is deeply nourishing for the soul.

How Heat Therapy Complements the Other Stages

As we have explored throughout this book, the Reset Way is founded on the principle of synergy – the idea that the whole is greater than the sum of its parts. Each stage of the reset protocol, from compression to cold plunge, works in harmony with the others to create a powerful, holistic approach to health and well-being. The jacuzzi, with its emphasis on heat therapy and relaxation, plays a vital role in this synergistic dance.

On a physiological level, the heat of the jacuzzi can help to amplify and extend the benefits of the other stages. For example, the increased blood flow and reduced inflammation promoted by the sauna can be further enhanced by the targeted massage and buoyancy of the jacuzzi. Similarly, the metabolic boost and fat-burning effects of cold plunge can be complemented by the gentle, sustained heat of the jacuzzi, helping to keep the body in a state of heightened calorie burn and detoxification.

On a psychological level, the deep relaxation and stress relief offered by the jacuzzi can help to counterbalance the intense, stimulating effects of tools like compression and red light therapy. By providing a space for quiet introspection and release, the jacuzzi can help to regulate the nervous system, promote emotional equilibrium, and support overall mental health and resilience.

Ultimately, the power of the jacuzzi lies in its ability to nourish and restore the body and mind in a way that is both deeply comforting and profoundly transformative. By making heat therapy and relaxation a regular part of your reset routine, you can tap into a boundless source of healing and rejuvenation that elevates and enhances the benefits of the other stages.

Maximizing Relaxation and Recovery in the Jacuzzi

To fully harness the potential of the jacuzzi, it is important to approach your sessions with intention, mindfulness, and a spirit of self-care. Here are a few tips to help you maximize the relaxation and recovery benefits of your jacuzzi time:

1. Set the Scene–Create a soothing, inviting environment by adjusting the lighting, music, and temperature to your liking. Consider adding elements like candles, essential oils, or soft towels to enhance the sensory experience and promote deeper relaxation.

2. Breathe Deeply–As you settle into the warm water, take a few deep, slow breaths, allowing your body to release any tension

or tightness. Focus on the sensation of the water against your skin, the gentle massage of the jets, and the quiet stillness of the moment.

3. Stay Hydrated–The heat of the jacuzzi can be dehydrating, so be sure to drink plenty of water before, during, and after your sessions. Consider keeping a cool glass of water or herbal tea nearby to sip on as you soak.

4. Use Mindful Movement–While the jacuzzi is primarily a place for stillness and relaxation, gentle stretching and movement can help to enhance circulation, release tension, and promote a deeper sense of body awareness. Experiment with slow, mindful movements like neck rolls, shoulder shrugs, and gentle twists to help your body fully unwind.

5. Practice Gratitude–As you bask in the warmth and comfort of the jacuzzi, take a moment to reflect on the many blessings in your life. Cultivating a sense of gratitude and appreciation can help to deepen the relaxation response and promote a greater sense of overall well-being.

By approaching your jacuzzi sessions with presence, care, and a spirit of self-love, you can transform this simple tool into a powerful catalyst for healing, growth, and transformation. As we come to the end of our exploration of the Reset Way, the jacuzzi stands as a testament to the power of small, intentional practices to create profound shifts in our health and happiness. So embrace the warmth, surrender to the moment, and let the transformative potential of the jacuzzi work its magic on your body, mind, and soul.

References

1. Kuczera, M., & Kokot, F. (1996). The influence of warm bath on the blood pressure in healthy and hypertensive subjects. Zentralblatt fur Gynakologie, 118(8), 447-451.
2. Becker, B. E. (2009). Aquatic therapy: scientific foundations and clinical rehabilitation applications. PM&R, 1(9), 859-872.
3. Goto, Y., Hayasaka, S., Kurihara, S., & Nakamura, Y. (2018). Physical and mental effects of bathing: a randomized intervention study. Evidence-Based Complementary and Alternative Medicine, 2018, 9521086.
4. An, J., Lee, I., & Yi, Y. (2019). The thermal effects of water immersion on health outcomes: an integrative review. International Journal of Environmental Research and Public Health, 16(7), 1280.

Part III: Implementing the Reset Way

Chapter 9: Creating Your Personal Reset Routine

As we have explored throughout this book, the Reset Way offers a powerful framework for optimizing health, vitality, and overall well-being. By integrating a range of science-backed tools and practices, from compression and red light therapy to sauna and cold plunge, we can tap into our body's innate healing potential and unlock new levels of energy, resilience, and joy. However, the true magic of the Reset Way lies not in any one tool or technique, but in the personalized application of these principles to your unique needs, goals, and lifestyle.

In this chapter, we will guide you through the process of creating your own customized reset routine. We will start by helping you assess your current state of health and well-being, identify your core wellness goals, and pinpoint any specific challenges or obstacles you may be facing. From there, we will explore how to tailor the 5-stage reset protocol to your individual needs, taking into account factors such as time constraints, personal preferences, and accessibility. Finally, we will offer practical strategies for seamlessly integrating your reset routine into your daily or weekly schedule, so that you can make this transformative practice a sustainable and enjoyable part of your life.

Whether you are a busy professional, a dedicated athlete, a caring parent, or simply someone seeking to live their best life, this chapter will provide you with the tools and insights you need to design a reset routine that works for you. So let's dive in and start crafting your personal roadmap to optimal health and happiness.

Assessing Your Current Lifestyle and Wellness Goals

The first step in creating your personalized reset routine is to take stock of your current state of health and well-being. This involves not only assessing your physical symptoms and challenges, but also examining your mental, emotional, and spiritual landscape. Some key questions to ask yourself might include:

1. How would I rate my overall energy levels and vitality on a scale of 1-10?

2. What are my biggest sources of stress or anxiety, and how are they impacting my health?

3. Do I have any chronic pain, inflammation, or other physical symptoms that are holding me back?

4. How satisfied am I with my current fitness level, body composition, and athletic performance?

5. What are my sleep patterns like, and do I wake up feeling rested and refreshed?

6. How would I describe my relationship with food and nutrition, and are there any changes I would like to make?

7. What brings me joy and fulfillment, and how can I incorporate more of these activities into my life?

By honestly and thoughtfully reflecting on these questions, you can start to build a clear picture of your current wellness landscape and identify any areas that may benefit from targeted support and attention.

Next, it's important to get clear on your specific wellness goals and aspirations. What does optimal health and happiness look like for you? Do you want to have more energy and vitality to keep up with your busy lifestyle? Are you seeking relief from chronic pain or inflammation? Do you want to improve your athletic performance or body composition? Or are you simply looking to cultivate a greater sense of balance, peace, and joy in your life?

Whatever your goals may be, it's important to make them specific, measurable, and achievable. Rather than setting a vague intention to "get healthy," for example, you might set a goal to "increase my energy levels by 25% and reduce my inflammation markers by 50% over the next three months." By defining your goals in concrete terms, you can create a clear roadmap for your reset journey and track your progress along the way.

Tailoring the 5-Stage Reset to Your Needs

Once you have a clear understanding of your current state of health and your specific wellness goals, the next step is to tailor the 5-stage reset protocol to your individual needs and preferences. While the basic framework of compression, red light therapy, sauna, cold plunge, and jacuzzi remains constant, there is plenty of room for customization and adaptation within each stage.

For example, if you have limited time or access to specialized equipment, you might focus on incorporating more accessible tools like compression socks, portable red light devices, and contrast showers into your routine. On the other hand, if you have a dedicated home gym or access to a full-service wellness center, you might opt for more advanced modalities like pneumatic compression boots, infrared saunas, and cold plunge pools.

Similarly, the duration, frequency, and intensity of each stage can be adjusted based on your individual tolerance, preferences, and goals. If you are new to cold exposure, for example, you might start with just 30 seconds of cold shower at the end of a warm shower, and gradually work your way up to longer and colder sessions over time. If you are an experienced sauna user, you might experiment with higher temperatures, longer durations, or the addition of aromatherapy or guided meditation to deepen the benefits.

Ultimately, the key is to find a balance that challenges you without overwhelming you, and that fits seamlessly into your existing lifestyle and routines. By listening to your body, honoring your preferences, and being willing to experiment and adapt, you can create a personalized reset protocol that is both effective and enjoyable.

Integrating the Reset into Your Daily or Weekly Schedule

Once you have tailored the 5-stage reset to your individual needs and preferences, the final step is to integrate this transformative practice into your daily or weekly schedule. This is where the rubber meets the road, and where many people can struggle to maintain consistency and momentum over time.

One of the keys to successful integration is to start small and build gradually. Rather than trying to overhaul your entire lifestyle overnight, focus on incorporating one or two reset elements into your existing routine, and then gradually adding more as you build confidence and momentum. For example, you might start by adding a 10-minute red light therapy session to your morning routine, or ending your daily shower with a 30-second blast of cold water.

Another important strategy is to anchor your reset practices to existing habits or routines. By piggy-backing on behaviors that are already automatic and ingrained, you can reduce the mental effort and willpower required to maintain your reset practice. For example, you might do a few minutes of compression therapy while watching your favorite TV show in the evening, or hop into the sauna for a quick sweat session right after your weekly gym workout.

It can also be helpful to enlist the support and accountability of others, whether that means joining a local wellness community, working with a coach or therapist, or simply sharing your goals and progress with friends and loved ones. By surrounding yourself with people who share your values and aspirations, you can tap into a powerful source of motivation, inspiration, and encouragement.

Ultimately, the key to successful integration is to approach your reset practice with a spirit of curiosity, experimentation, and self-compassion. There will inevitably be days when you fall short of your goals or struggle to maintain momentum, and that's okay. The Reset Way is not about perfection, but about progress – about taking small, consistent steps towards greater health, happiness, and vitality, one day at a time.

By following the strategies outlined in this chapter – assessing your current state of health, setting clear and specific wellness goals, tailoring the 5-stage reset to your individual needs, and integrating this transformative practice into your daily or weekly routine – you can create a personalized reset routine that is both effective and sustainable. And as you begin to experience the profound benefits of this holistic approach to health and well-being, you may find that your reset practice becomes not just a part of your life, but a way of life – a powerful tool for unlocking your full potential and living your best life, each and every day.

References

1. Prochaska, J. O., & Velicer, W. F. (1997). The transtheoretical model of health behavior change. American Journal of Health Promotion, 12(1), 38-48.
2. Gardner, B., Lally, P., & Wardle, J. (2012). Making health habitual: the psychology of 'habit-formation' and general practice. British Journal of General Practice, 62(605), 664-666.
3. Oettingen, G., & Gollwitzer, P. M. (2010). Strategies of setting and implementing goals. In J. E. Maddux & J. P. Tangney (Eds.), Social Psychological Foundations of Clinical Psychology (pp. 114-135). The Guilford Press.
4. Goyal, M., Singh, S., Sibinga, E. M., Gould, N. F., Rowland-Seymour, A., Sharma, R., ... & Haythornthwaite, J. A. (2014). Meditation programs for psychological stress and well-being: a systematic review and meta-analysis. JAMA Internal Medicine, 174(3), 357-368.

Chapter 10: Complementary Practices for Optimal Results

As we have seen throughout this book, the Reset Way offers a comprehensive approach to health and well-being, integrating a range of powerful tools and techniques to support the body's natural healing processes. From the targeted benefits of compression and red light therapy to the rejuvenating effects of sauna, cold plunge, and jacuzzi, each stage of the reset protocol works synergistically to promote optimal physical, mental, and emotional wellness. However, to truly maximize the transformative potential of the Reset Way, it is important to extend these principles beyond the core 5-stage protocol and into other areas of your life.

In this chapter, we will explore a range of complementary practices that can amplify and sustain the benefits of your reset routine. We will start by examining the crucial role of nutrition and hydration in supporting your body's natural detoxification and healing processes. From there, we will delve into the importance of sleep and stress management in promoting resilience, recovery, and overall well-being. Finally, we will explore the transformative power of mindfulness and meditation as tools for cultivating greater awareness, presence, and inner peace.

By integrating these complementary practices into your daily life, you can create a powerful synergy with your core reset routine, supporting your body and mind from every angle and unlocking new levels of vitality, resilience, and joy. So let's dive in and explore the holistic path to optimal health and happiness.

Nutrition and Hydration Tips

The foundation of any successful wellness program is a nutrient-dense, whole-foods based diet that provides your body with the raw materials it needs to thrive. When it comes to optimizing the benefits of your reset routine, there are a few key nutritional strategies to keep in mind:

1. Prioritize anti-inflammatory foods: Chronic inflammation is at the root of many chronic diseases and can significantly impair your body's ability to heal and recover. To combat inflammation, focus on incorporating plenty of anti-inflammatory foods into your diet, such as leafy greens, berries, fatty fish, nuts, and seeds. At the same time, minimize your intake of pro-inflammatory foods, such as refined carbohydrates, processed meats, and trans fats.

2. Support detoxification pathways: Your body is equipped with a complex system of detoxification pathways that help to neutralize and eliminate harmful toxins and metabolic waste products. To support these pathways, focus on incorporating plenty of cruciferous vegetables (such as broccoli, kale, and Brussels sprouts), which are rich in sulfur-containing compounds that aid in detoxification. Other detox-supportive foods include garlic, onions, turmeric, and citrus fruits.

3. Stay well-hydrated: Proper hydration is essential for virtually every aspect of health, from digestion and nutrient absorption to cognitive function and physical performance. When it comes to your reset routine, staying well-hydrated is particularly important for supporting lymphatic flow, flushing out toxins, and maintaining optimal circulation. Aim to drink at least half your body weight in ounces of water each day, and consider incorporating hydrating foods like cucumbers, melons, and zucchini into your diet as well.

4. Time your meals strategically: The timing of your meals can have a significant impact on your body's ability to absorb and utilize nutrients. In general, it is best to consume your largest meals earlier in the day, when your digestive fire is strongest,

and to avoid eating heavy, hard-to-digest foods late at night. If you are incorporating fasting or time-restricted eating into your reset routine, be sure to break your fast with a nutrient-dense, easily digestible meal to support your body's natural healing processes.

By following these nutritional strategies and staying well-hydrated throughout the day, you can create a strong foundation for your reset routine and support your body's natural ability to heal, detoxify, and thrive.

The Role of Sleep and Stress Management

In addition to nutrition and hydration, sleep and stress management are two of the most important complementary practices for optimizing the benefits of your reset routine. When it comes to health and well-being, sleep and stress are two sides of the same coin – both are essential for recovery, repair, and resilience, and both can have a profound impact on your physical, mental, and emotional state.

On the sleep front, aim to get at least 7-9 hours of high-quality, uninterrupted sleep each night. This means creating a sleep environment that is cool, dark, and quiet, and avoiding stimulating activities (such as screen time or intense exercise) in the hours leading up to bedtime. You may also want to experiment with sleep-supportive practices such as meditation, deep breathing, or progressive muscle relaxation to help you unwind and drift off more easily.

When it comes to stress management, the key is to find practices that help you cultivate a sense of calm, resilience, and inner peace in the face of life's challenges. This might include techniques such as deep breathing, yoga, tai chi, or spending time in nature. It could also involve more structured stress-management practices such as cognitive-behavioral therapy or mindfulness-based stress reduction.

Ultimately, the goal is to create a holistic approach to stress management that addresses both the physical and emotional aspects of stress. By incorporating practices that help you relax your body, quiet your mind, and connect with your inner wisdom and resilience, you can create a powerful buffer against the negative effects of stress and support your overall health and well-being.

Incorporating Mindfulness and Meditation

Finally, no discussion of complementary practices for optimal health would be complete without touching on the transformative power of mindfulness and meditation. At its core, mindfulness is the practice of bringing your full attention and awareness to the present moment, without judgment or resistance. By cultivating this kind of open, curious, and accepting attitude towards your experience, you can begin to release the grip of stress, anxiety, and other negative mental and emotional states, and tap into a deeper sense of peace, clarity, and well-being.

One of the most powerful ways to cultivate mindfulness is through the practice of meditation. Whether you prefer guided visualizations, silent contemplation, or movement-based practices like yoga or tai chi, the key is to find a meditation style that resonates with you and to make it a regular part of your daily routine.

When it comes to incorporating meditation into your reset routine, there are a few key strategies to keep in mind. First, start small and build gradually. Even just a few minutes of meditation each day can have a profound impact on your mental and emotional state, so don't feel like you need to sit for hours on end to experience the benefits.

Second, find a meditation space that feels calm, peaceful, and conducive to relaxation. This might be a quiet corner of your home, a local park or nature reserve, or even a dedicated meditation studio or retreat center.

Finally, approach your meditation practice with a spirit of curiosity, openness, and self-compassion. Remember that meditation is not about achieving a particular state of mind or eliminating all thoughts and distractions, but rather about cultivating a more accepting and compassionate relationship with your own experience.

By incorporating mindfulness and meditation into your daily routine, you can tap into a powerful source of inner peace, clarity, and resilience that can support and amplify the benefits of your reset practice. Whether you are new to meditation or a seasoned practitioner, the key is to approach this practice with a beginner's mind, a willingness to explore, and a deep commitment to your own health and well-being.

As we come to the end of this chapter on complementary practices for optimal health, it is important to remember that true wellness is not a destination, but a journey – a lifelong process of learning, growth, and self-discovery. By integrating nutrition, hydration, sleep, stress management, mindfulness, and meditation into your daily life, you can create a strong foundation for your reset practice and support your body, mind, and spirit in reaching their fullest potential. So embrace the journey, trust the process, and know that with each small step, you are moving closer to the vibrant, joyful, and resilient life you deserve.

References

1. Lopresti, A. L., Hood, S. D., & Drummond, P. D. (2013). A review of lifestyle factors that contribute to important pathways associated with major depression: diet, sleep and exercise. Journal of Affective Disorders, 148(1), 12-27.
2. Black, D. S., & Slavich, G. M. (2016). Mindfulness meditation and the immune system: a systematic review of randomized controlled trials. Annals of the New York Academy of Sciences, 1373(1), 13-24.
3. Irwin, M. R. (2015). Why sleep is important for health: a psychoneuroimmunology perspective. Annual Review of Psychology, 66, 143-172.
4. Khalsa, S. B. S. (2004). Treatment of chronic insomnia with yoga: A preliminary study with sleep–wake diaries. Applied Psychophysiology and Biofeedback, 29(4), 269-278.

Chapter 11: Transforming Your Life with the Reset Way

As we have explored throughout this book, the Reset Way offers a powerful and transformative approach to health and well-being, one that can help you unlock your full potential and live your best life. By integrating the core principles of compression, red light therapy, sauna, cold plunge, and jacuzzi with complementary practices like nutrition, hydration, sleep, stress management, and mindfulness, you can create a holistic and synergistic approach to wellness that supports your body, mind, and spirit from every angle.

But don't just take our word for it – the true power of the Reset Way lies in the real-life stories of transformation and success that have emerged from this approach. In this chapter, we will share some of these inspiring stories, highlighting the profound and lasting impact that the Reset Way has had on people's lives. From there, we will explore the long-term benefits of adopting this approach, including improved physical health, mental clarity, emotional resilience, and overall quality of life. Finally, we will offer practical strategies for overcoming common challenges and staying motivated on your reset journey, so that you can sustain the benefits of this transformative practice for years to come.

Whether you are just starting out on your wellness journey or are a seasoned practitioner looking to take your health to the next level, this chapter will provide you with the inspiration, guidance, and tools you need to transform your life with the Reset Way. So let's dive in and discover the incredible possibilities that await you.

Real-Life Success Stories

One of the most powerful testaments to the transformative potential of the Reset Way comes from the real-life stories of individuals who have experienced its benefits firsthand. Take, for example, the story of Sarah, a 45-year-old mother of three who had been struggling with chronic fatigue, digestive issues, and anxiety for years. Despite trying countless diets, supplements, and therapies, nothing seemed to provide lasting relief – until she discovered the Reset Way.

By incorporating regular compression therapy, red light therapy, and sauna sessions into her weekly routine, Sarah began to notice a significant improvement in her energy levels and overall sense of well-being. She also found that the mindfulness and stress-management techniques she learned through the Reset Way helped her to feel more grounded, centered, and resilient in the face of life's challenges.

Another inspiring story comes from Mark, a 55-year-old executive who had been struggling with high blood pressure, weight gain, and poor sleep for decades. After hearing about the Reset Way from a colleague, Mark decided to give it a try – and was amazed by the results. Within just a few weeks of incorporating cold plunge therapy and strategic nutrition into his daily routine, Mark began to notice a significant improvement in his blood pressure, body composition, and sleep quality. He also found that the increased mental clarity and focus he experienced through the Reset Way helped him to be more productive and effective in his work and personal life.

These are just a few examples of the many success stories that have emerged from the Reset Way. From athletes and entrepreneurs to stay-at-home parents and retirees, people from all walks of life have experienced the transformative benefits of this holistic approach to health and well-being.

Long-Term Benefits of Adopting the Reset Approach

While the immediate benefits of the Reset Way can be profound, the true power of this approach lies in its ability to create lasting, sustainable changes in your health and well-being. By making the Reset Way a consistent part of your lifestyle, you can experience a wide range of long-term benefits, including:

1. Improved physical health: Regular practice of the Reset Way can help to support cardiovascular health, boost immune function, improve muscle tone and flexibility, and reduce the risk of chronic diseases like obesity, diabetes, and heart disease.

2. Enhanced mental clarity and focus: The combination of physical and mental practices in the Reset Way can help to improve cognitive function, increase mental clarity and focus, and reduce the risk of age-related cognitive decline.

3. Greater emotional resilience: By incorporating stress-management and mindfulness techniques into your daily routine, you can cultivate greater emotional resilience and adaptability, helping you to navigate life's challenges with greater ease and grace.

4. Increased energy and vitality: The synergistic effects of the Reset Way can help to boost your overall energy and vitality, allowing you to show up more fully and effectively in all areas of your life.

5. Improved quality of life: Ultimately, the greatest benefit of the Reset Way is its ability to enhance your overall quality of life. By supporting your physical, mental, and emotional well-being, this approach can help you to live a more joyful, fulfilling, and purposeful life, one that is aligned with your deepest values and aspirations.

Overcoming Challenges and Staying Motivated

Of course, like any transformative journey, the path of the Reset Way is not always easy. Along the way, you may encounter challenges, setbacks, and obstacles that test your resolve and commitment to this practice. However, by staying focused on your goals, cultivating a supportive community, and developing a toolkit of motivational strategies, you can overcome these challenges and sustain the benefits of the Reset Way for the long haul.

One key strategy for staying motivated is to connect with a community of like-minded individuals who share your passion for health and wellness. Whether you join a local Reset Way group, participate in online forums or social media communities, or simply enlist the support of friends and family members, having a network of people to share your journey with can provide a powerful source of inspiration, accountability, and encouragement.

Another important strategy is to set clear, achievable goals for your Reset Way practice, and to celebrate your progress along the way. Whether your goal is to complete a certain number of sauna sessions per week, maintain a consistent meditation practice, or simply feel more energized and vibrant each day, having a clear target to work towards can help you stay focused and motivated.

Finally, it is important to approach your Reset Way journey with a spirit of self-compassion and patience. Remember that transformation is a process, not an event, and that setbacks and challenges are a natural part of any journey of growth and self-discovery. By treating yourself with kindness and understanding, and by trusting in the wisdom and resilience of your body and mind, you can weather any storm and emerge stronger, more vibrant, and more fully alive.

As we come to the end of this book, we hope that you feel inspired and empowered to embark on your own Reset Way journey. Whether you are a seasoned wellness warrior or a curious beginner, the principles and practices outlined in these pages offer a powerful roadmap for unlocking your full potential and living your best life. So take a deep breath, trust in the process, and know that with each small step, you are moving closer to the vibrant, joyful, and resilient life you deserve. The Reset Way is not just a practice – it is a path, a journey, and a way of being in the world. May it guide you, support you, and transform you, now and always.

References

1. Buettner, D. (2012). The Blue Zones: 9 Lessons for Living Longer from the People Who've Lived the Longest. National Geographic Books.
2. Williamson, G. (2016). The Longevity Diet: Discover the New Science Behind Stem Cell Activation and Regeneration to Slow Aging, Fight Disease, and Optimize Weight. Harmony.
3. Lipton, B. H. (2015). The Biology of Belief: Unleashing the Power of Consciousness, Matter, and Miracles. Hay House.
4. Sinclair, D. A., & LaPlante, M. D. (2019). Lifespan: Why We Age—and Why We Don't Have To. Atria Books.

Conclusion

As we come to the end of our exploration of the Reset Way, it is clear that this holistic approach to health and well-being offers a powerful and transformative path for anyone seeking to unlock their full potential and live their best life. By integrating a range of science-backed tools and techniques, from compression therapy and red light therapy to sauna, cold plunge, and jacuzzi, the Reset Way provides a comprehensive framework for supporting the body's natural healing processes and promoting optimal physical, mental, and emotional wellness.

At the heart of the Reset Way lies a set of core principles that guide and inform every aspect of this approach. These principles include a deep respect for the body's innate wisdom and resilience, a commitment to self-care and self-discovery, and a recognition of the interconnectedness of all aspects of our being. By aligning ourselves with these principles and incorporating them into our daily lives, we can create a strong foundation for lasting health, happiness, and vitality.

Recap of the Key Principles of the Reset Way

Throughout this book, we have explored the key principles that underlie the Reset Way, and how they can be applied to create a personalized and effective wellness routine. These principles include:

1. Synergy: The Reset Way recognizes that true health and well-being emerge from the synergistic interplay of multiple factors, including physical, mental, emotional, and spiritual well-being. By addressing all of these aspects of our being in a holistic and integrated way, we can create a powerful catalyst for healing and transformation.

2. Individuality: While the Reset Way offers a comprehensive framework for health and wellness, it also recognizes that

each person's needs and preferences are unique. By tailoring the various tools and techniques of the Reset Way to our individual constitution, lifestyle, and goals, we can create a personalized approach that works for us on every level.

3. Consistency: The benefits of the Reset Way are cumulative and synergistic, meaning that the more consistently we incorporate these practices into our daily lives, the more profound and lasting the results will be. By making the Reset Way a non-negotiable part of our routine, we can create a powerful momentum for positive change and transformation.

4. Mindfulness: The Reset Way is not just about the specific tools and techniques we use, but also about the quality of awareness and presence we bring to our practice. By approaching our wellness journey with a spirit of mindfulness, curiosity, and self-compassion, we can deepen our understanding of ourselves and cultivate a more harmonious and fulfilling relationship with our body, mind, and spirit.

By keeping these principles at the forefront of our mind and integrating them into every aspect of our Reset Way practice, we can create a strong and resilient foundation for optimal health and well-being.

Encouragement for Readers to Embrace Self-Care and Wellness

One of the most important messages of the Reset Way is that true health and happiness are not something that can be passively received or externally imposed, but rather must be actively cultivated and nurtured from within. This means taking responsibility for our own well-being, and making self-care a non-negotiable priority in our lives.

For many of us, this can be a challenging and even daunting prospect. In a world that often prioritizes productivity, achievement, and external validation over internal well-being, it can be easy to neglect or dismiss our own needs and desires. We may feel guilty or selfish for taking time for ourselves, or worry that we are not deserving of the care and attention we need to thrive.

However, the truth is that self-care is not a luxury or an indulgence, but rather a fundamental necessity for anyone seeking to live a healthy, happy, and fulfilling life. When we prioritize our own well-being and make space for practices that nourish and support us on every level, we not only benefit ourselves, but also everyone around us. We show up more fully and authentically in our relationships, our work, and our communities, and we inspire others to do the same.

So if you take one message from this book, let it be this: you are worthy of self-care, and your well-being matters. By embracing the principles and practices of the Reset Way, you are not only investing in your own health and happiness, but also contributing to the greater well-being of the world around you. Every small step you take towards self-care and self-discovery ripples out into the world, creating a powerful wave of positive change and transformation.

The Potential for Profound Personal Transformation

Ultimately, the Reset Way is about much more than just feeling better or looking better – it is about discovering and expressing the fullest and most authentic version of ourselves. By committing to this holistic and transformative approach to wellness, we open ourselves up to a profound journey of personal growth and self-discovery, one that can reshape every aspect of our lives.

As we incorporate the various tools and techniques of the Reset Way into our daily routine, we begin to experience a range of benefits that go far beyond the physical. We may find that we have more energy, clarity, and focus, and that we are better able to manage stress and navigate challenges with resilience and grace. We may also discover new depths of creativity, intuition, and spiritual connection, as we learn to trust and listen to the wisdom of our body and soul.

Over time, these benefits can compound and synergize, leading to a profound transformation in our overall quality of life. We may find that we are more joyful, present, and engaged in our relationships, our work, and our passions. We may also experience a deeper sense of purpose and meaning, as we align ourselves with our true values and desires and create a life that truly reflects who we are.

Of course, this transformation is not always easy or linear. Like any journey of growth and self-discovery, the path of the Reset Way will inevitably involve challenges, setbacks, and moments of doubt or resistance. However, by staying committed to the process and trusting in the wisdom and resilience of our own being, we can weather these storms and emerge stronger, wiser, and more fully alive.

As we come to the end of this book, we invite you to embrace the potential for profound personal transformation that the Reset Way offers. Whether you are a seasoned wellness warrior or a curious beginner, the principles and practices outlined in these pages can help you unlock your full potential and create a life of vibrant health, authentic happiness, and limitless possibility.

So take a deep breath, trust in the journey, and know that with each small step, you are moving closer to the radiant, resilient, and truly amazing being you were born to be. The Reset Way is not a destination, but a path – a way of living, learning, and growing that can support and inspire you for a lifetime. May it be a source of strength, guidance, and transformation for you, now and always.

References

1. Neff, K. D., & Germer, C. K. (2013). A pilot study and randomized controlled trial of the mindful self-compassion program. Journal of Clinical Psychology, 69(1), 28-44.
2. Perlmutter, D. (2020). Brain Wash: Detox Your Mind for Clearer Thinking, Deeper Relationships, and Lasting Happiness. Little, Brown Spark.
3. Dispenza, J. (2014). You Are the Placebo: Making Your Mind Matter. Hay House.
4. Hanson, R. (2013). Hardwiring Happiness: The New Brain Science of Contentment, Calm, and Confidence. Harmony.

Appendices

As you embark on your Reset Way journey, you may find yourself seeking additional resources, information, and support to help you deepen your practice and maximize the benefits of this transformative approach to health and well-being. In this final section of the book, we have compiled a range of appendices designed to provide you with the tools, insights, and inspiration you need to take your Reset Way experience to the next level.

Whether you are looking for guidance on finding reset facilities or equipment, seeking to expand your knowledge through recommended reading and references, or simply want to clarify your understanding of key terms and concepts, these appendices offer a wealth of valuable information and support.

Resources for Finding Reset Facilities or Equipment

One of the most common questions we receive from readers is how to find quality reset facilities or equipment in their local area. While the specific availability of these resources may vary depending on your location, there are a number of strategies you can use to locate and access the tools and spaces you need to support your Reset Way practice.

One of the first places to start is by searching online for wellness centers, spas, or fitness facilities that offer the specific modalities you are interested in, such as compression therapy, red light therapy, sauna, cold plunge, or jacuzzi. Many of these facilities will have websites or social media pages that provide detailed information about their services, pricing, and availability.

Another great resource is to connect with local wellness communities or groups, either online or in person. These communities can be a wealth of information and support, offering recommendations for trusted providers, sharing personal experiences and insights, and even organizing group events or outings to reset facilities.

If you are interested in purchasing your own reset equipment for home use, there are a number of reputable suppliers and manufacturers that offer high-quality products designed specifically for personal wellness. From portable red light therapy devices and compression boots to inflatable saunas and cold plunge tubs, these products can offer a convenient and cost-effective way to incorporate the Reset Way into your daily routine.

Ultimately, the key to finding the right reset facilities or equipment for your needs is to do your research, ask for recommendations, and trust your instincts. By taking the time to explore your options and invest in quality resources, you can create a powerful and sustainable foundation for your Reset Way practice.

Recommended Reading and References

In addition to the information and insights provided in this book, there are countless other resources available for those seeking to deepen their understanding of the science, philosophy, and practice of the Reset Way. Here are just a few of our top recommendations for further reading and exploration:

- "The Biology of Belief" by Bruce Lipton–This groundbreaking book explores the connection between mind and matter, and how our thoughts and beliefs can influence our physical health and well-being.

- "The Wim Hof Method" by Wim Hof–Written by the renowned Dutch athlete and extreme athlete, this book offers a comprehensive guide to cold therapy and breathwork, and how these practices can be used to optimize health, performance, and resilience.

- "The Miracle Morning" by Hal Elrod–This popular self-help book provides a simple and effective framework for creating a powerful morning routine that can transform every aspect of your life, from your health and relationships to your career and personal growth.

- "The Science of Yoga" by William J. Broad–This thoroughly researched and engaging book explores the history, philosophy, and science behind the practice of yoga, and how this ancient tradition can be adapted and applied for modern health and well-being.

- "The Telomere Effect" by Elizabeth Blackburn and Elissa Epel–Written by two leading experts in the field of aging and longevity, this book explores the role of telomeres in the aging process, and how lifestyle factors like stress, diet, and exercise can influence the length and health of these vital DNA structures.

Of course, these are just a few examples of the many excellent resources available on the topics of health, wellness, and personal transformation. We encourage you to explore these and other books, articles, and resources that resonate with your interests and goals, and to use them as a springboard for your own learning and growth.

Glossary of Key Terms

Finally, to help clarify and reinforce your understanding of the key concepts and terminology used throughout this book, we have compiled a glossary of important terms related to the Reset Way and its various tools and techniques.

- **Autonomic Nervous System**–The part of the nervous system responsible for regulating involuntary body functions, such as heart rate, digestion, and respiratory rate.

- **Brown Adipose Tissue (BAT)**–A type of metabolically active fat tissue that helps regulate body temperature and energy expenditure.

- **Cardiovascular System**–The system of the body that includes the heart, blood vessels, and blood, and is responsible for circulating oxygen and nutrients throughout the body.

- **Circadian Rhythm**–The natural 24-hour cycle of physiological processes in the body, including the sleep-wake cycle, hormone production, and body temperature regulation.

- **Cold Plunge**–The practice of immersing the body in cold water for short periods of time, typically between 30 seconds and several minutes, in order to stimulate physiological and psychological benefits.

- **Compression Therapy**–The use of compression garments or devices to apply controlled pressure to the limbs, in order to promote circulation, reduce swelling, and support recovery.

- **Heat Shock Proteins (HSPs)**–A family of proteins produced by cells in response to stressors such as heat, cold, or oxidative stress, which help to protect and repair cellular structures.

- **Homeostasis**–The tendency of the body to maintain a stable internal environment, despite changes in the external environment.

- **Hydrotherapy**–The use of water for therapeutic purposes, including baths, showers, and other forms of immersion or application.

- **Hyperthermia**–An abnormally high body temperature, often induced therapeutically through practices such as sauna or hot water immersion.

- **Hypothalamic-Pituitary-Adrenal (HPA) Axis**–The complex system of feedback interactions between the hypothalamus, pituitary gland, and adrenal glands that regulates the body's response to stress.

- **Lymphatic System**–The network of tissues, vessels, and organs that helps to maintain fluid balance, fight infection, and remove cellular waste products from the body.

- **Mindfulness**–The practice of bringing one's attention to the present moment, with openness, curiosity, and non-judgment.

- **Mitochondria**–The energy-producing organelles found in every cell of the body, responsible for converting nutrients into usable energy in the form of ATP.

- **Photobiomodulation**–The use of light, typically in the red or near-infrared spectrum, to stimulate cellular and physiological processes in the body.

- **Polyvagal Theory**–A model of the autonomic nervous system that emphasizes the role of the vagus nerve in regulating physiological and emotional states.

- **Prana**–A term used in Ayurvedic and yogic traditions to refer to the vital life force energy that animates all living beings.

- **Proprioception**–The sense of the position and movement of the body, including the sense of effort, force, and heaviness.

- **Qi**–A term used in Traditional Chinese Medicine to refer to the vital life force energy that flows through the body and regulates physiological and emotional processes.

- **Red Light Therapy**–The use of red and near-infrared light to stimulate cellular processes, reduce inflammation, and promote healing.

- **Telomeres**–The protective caps at the ends of chromosomes, which shorten with each cell division and are associated with the aging process.

- **Vagus Nerve**–The longest and most complex cranial nerve, which plays a key role in regulating the autonomic nervous system and the body's relaxation response.

By familiarizing yourself with these and other key terms related to the Reset Way, you can deepen your understanding of the principles and practices that underlie this transformative approach to health and well-being.

As we come to the end of this book, we hope that these appendices have provided you with additional resources, insights, and clarity to support your Reset Way journey. Remember, the path to optimal health and happiness is an ongoing process of learning, growth, and self-discovery. By staying curious, committed, and open to new possibilities, you can continue to unlock the full potential of your mind, body, and spirit, and create a life of boundless vitality, joy, and fulfillment.

References

1. Huberman, A. D. (Host). (2021-present). Huberman Lab [Audio podcast]. https://hubermanlab.com/
2. Lipton, B. H. (2015). The Biology of Belief: Unleashing the Power of Consciousness, Matter, and Miracles. Hay House.
3. Hof, W. (2020). The Wim Hof Method: Activate Your Full Human Potential. Sounds True.
4. Elrod, H. (2012). The Miracle Morning: The Not-So-Obvious Secret Guaranteed to Transform Your Life (Before 8AM). Hal Elrod International, Inc.
5. Broad, W. J. (2012). The Science of Yoga: The Risks and the Rewards. Simon & Schuster.
6. Blackburn, E., & Epel, E. (2017). The Telomere Effect: A Revolutionary Approach to Living Younger, Healthier, Longer. Grand Central Publishing.